Aphrodite's
SECRETS

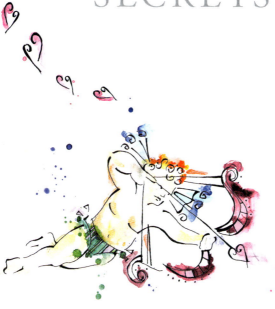

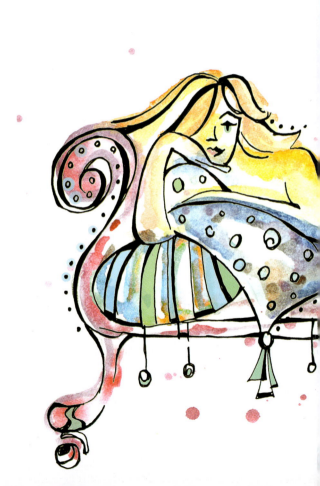

Aphrodite's SECRETS

DRESSING UP for
GETTING DOWN
and other ways to
UNLEASH your
inner SEX GODDESS

JOANNE E. BRUNN

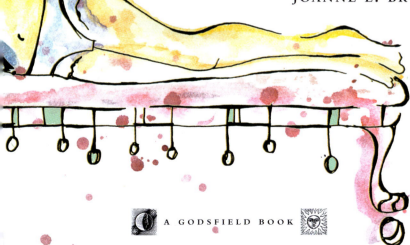

A GODSFIELD BOOK

Author dedication
To Aphrodite, for her continued inspiration in the art of love. To my husband, Lou Veltri, for his profound love, deep interest in who I am, and for being my muse for many of the suggestions in this book. To Brenda Rosen, for her encouragement during the writing process and her belief in me.

First published in Great Britain in 2004
by Godsfield Press Ltd,
Laurel House, Station Approach,
Alresford, Hampshire SO24 9JH, U.K.

www.godsfieldpress.com

Copyright © 2004 Godsfield Press
Text copyright © 2004 Joanne E. Brunn

Project Editor: Sarah Doughty
Illustrator: Anna Hunter-Downing
Project Designer: Ana Bjezancevic

Designed and produced for Godsfield Press
by The Bridgewater Book Company

All rights reserved. No part of this publication may be reproduced, stored in a retrieval system, or transmitted in any form or by any means, electronic, mechanical, photocopying, recording, or otherwise.

Joanne E. Brunn asserts the moral right to be identified as the author of this work.

10 9 8 7 6 5 4 3 2 1

Printed and bound in China

ISBN 1-84181-227-7

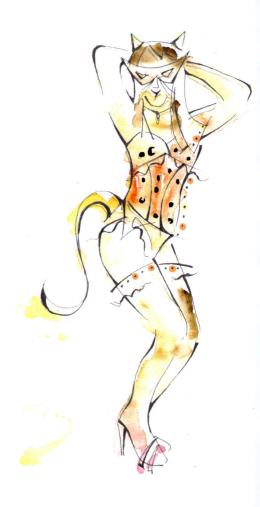

Contents

Unleashing Your Inner Love Goddess ♥♥♥♥♥♥♥ 6

A Thong of Love ♥♥♥♥♥♥♥ 12

Love Notes ♥♥♥♥♥♥♥ 24

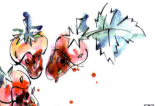

A Bath of Rose Petals ♥♥♥♥♥♥♥ 36

Dinner Delights ♥♥♥♥♥♥♥ 48

The Dance of the Veils ♥♥♥♥♥♥♥ 60

Body Painting Dessert ♥♥♥♥♥♥♥ 72

Pillow Talk ♥♥♥♥♥♥♥ 84

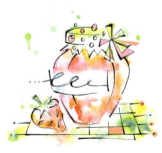

UNLEASHING YOUR INNER LOVE GODDESS

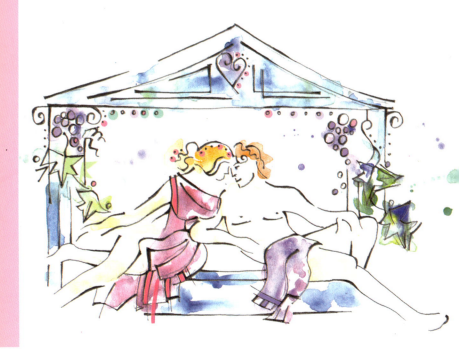

Love Goddess! What does this phrase evoke in you? If it makes you feel powerful and passionate, you probably already know all about your inner Love Goddess. If you feel frightened or skeptical, you may need some magical help to awaken a part of you that has been asleep way too long.

Do you think that only gods and goddesses or those air-brushed movie stars have magical powers? Hidden deep within you is all you need to know about love and magic. You know much more than you think you do about how to use your sensual prowess. And you can use that magic—imagination, creativity, zest, and a bit of naughtiness—to become a Love Goddess yourself. As the Sex and Love Goddess of all times, Aphrodite has some special tricks to share with you, along with ways to uncover what you already know. So get ready to have some fun and strut your magical stuff!

aphrodite's magic cestus

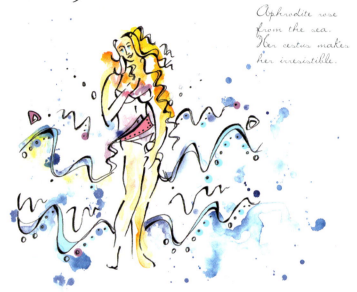

Aphrodite rose from the sea. Her cestus makes her irresistible.

Stories say that the secret of Aphrodite's charms was her golden embroidered *cestus*—a belt or scarf that had the power to make any man fall in love with her. When she wore her cestus, her seductive powers were so great that no god or mortal could resist her. All the great studs of the heavens like Hephestus the Smith, Mars the Warrior, and Hermes the Winged Messenger succumbed to her charms. Even the greatest god of all, Zeus himself, desired her. And as for mortal men, she couldn't keep Adonis away from her. Not that this was a problem, as he was quite the hottie, but a girl needs to rest sometimes! So be careful, and use your magic with caution and utmost discretion. After all, you want to choose the men who will fall at your feet.

You, too, can be irresistible to any man you desire. Really? Really! The secret of Aphrodite's magic cestus was really quite simple. When she wore it, she believed that no man could resist her. You see, in order to be a Love Goddess, you have to *believe* you're a Love Goddess. That's it. The rest happens quite naturally.

Read on and you'll see.

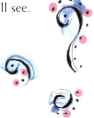

magical chant to invoke aphrodite

To enter into a Love Goddess state of mind, it's fun to evoke the essence of Aphrodite by honoring her with a chant. Remember to thank her for helping you out. You can do this as you are weaving your own magic cestus, taking a rose petal bath, seeking inspiration for a love message, or planning dinner or dessert for a special evening. In fact, you can offer her a chant any time you feel you need a little boost to get your love juices flowing.

Welcome the Love Goddess by honoring her with a chant.

❀

Welcome Aphrodite!

Goddess of Love, Goddess of Lust

Goddess of Beauty, Goddess of Marriage

Goddess of Fertility, Goddess of Laughter

Aphrodite—you are so many good things in one package

Let me in on your secrets.

You know how to turn a man's head with a wink of your eye

Your beauty is acknowledged by everyone

You are not afraid to go after what you want

You know how to soar to the heights of lovemaking

Your laughter sounds like sweet music

You are one extraordinary role model!

Please lend me a little of your magic tonight

I want to feel irresistible, ravishing, and enchanting

I want to say the right words at the right time

I want courage and confidence

I want to not burn the dinner or spill wine on my blouse!

Aphrodite, thanks for reminding me that I'm a Goddess too!

With you on my side and my magic cestus strapped on,

Nothing can stand in my way!

❀

A THONG OF LOVE

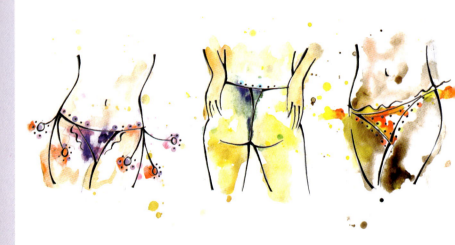

Dressing up for getting down can help bring a little of Aphrodite's love magic to your bedroom. Never underestimate the sex appeal of perfect undies. Ever since Aphrodite first buckled on her cestus (ancient Greek for "hot pants"), bedroom attire has been an important wardrobe item for every Love Goddess. Forget the boxers and go for something with a bit of lace or sparkles. What you're seeking is that special item that makes you feel ultrasexy when stripping off.

Shopping for your undies is part of the fun. Pick out a luscious pair (or maybe two or three). Make sure the color and design calls to you and that simply slipping them on makes you feel sexy and delicious. What's your undies' personality? Do flowers, ribbons, and silly prints reveal your girlish charms? Or maybe bold patterns and bright colors show that you're a girl who loves to laugh? Even a no-fuss, no-frills tomboy type can find undies that show off her mellow, laid back style. Your undies reveal the inner you, so shop carefully!

Or, for more magic, why not decorate your own?

knicker know-how

- ♥ Go wild picking out rhinestones, sequins, beads, baubles, or whatever decorations you fancy. Let your inner Love Goddess play with colors and shapes. Give yourself permission to be frivolous.
- ♥ Put on some music to set the mood, something with soft violin or flute if that's your preference, or maybe some sexy rhythm and blues or pounding trance music.
- ♥ Lay out your undies. Open your bags of rhinestones and sequins and sprinkle on the goodies in a random design. Think of the stars in the night sky. Let the Goddess in you guide your hand to create the perfect magical pattern. You can do no wrong.
- ♥ Don't worry about overdoing it. The more you glitter and sparkle and jingle and glow, the more irresistible you will be!
- ♥ Attach your design using fabric glue or needle and thread.
- ♥ You may wish to add sexy symbols or other motifs with fabric paint or glue glitter.

- ♥ Consider draping lace, ribbons, or strings of gems that will shimmy with your every movement.
- ♥ To add a bit of mystery, hang string beads around the leg openings.
- ♥ Consider other touches of your own. Perhaps add a fresh flower. Or anoint your undies with essential oils. Or add some personal jewelry.

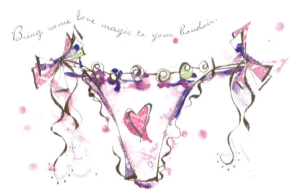

Bring some love magic to your boudoir.

- ♥ Stand back and admire your work. You have created your own magic cestus! Wearing these fancy pants, your seductive powers are so great that no man can resist you.

Go forth, Love Goddess, and conquer!

fab for fancy pants

If undies aren't your thing, you might want to create a magic T-shirt or bra or scarf. You can use all the same ideas as for the fancy pants. Pick out some wild colors, maybe some soft silks or velvets. Create spiral designs on your T-shirt with glue glitter or fabric paint. Hang strings of gems from your bra. Wrap ribbon around the straps. Glue sequins to your scarf. The wilder and crazier the better! Let your imagination soar! You get the idea.

The goal is to create something that makes you feel strong and sexy when you put it on. Something that screams "Love Goddess"!

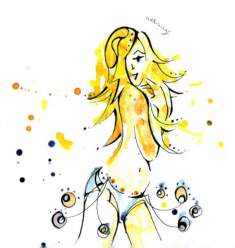

CUSTOMIZE YOUR UNDIES WITH THE FOLLOWING ITEMS:

- ♥ Fabric paint.
- ♥ Small bells.
- ♥ Sheer fabric to sew around the leg openings and tie at the ankle in a harem-pants style.
- ♥ Dried flowers.
- ♥ Jewelry.
- ♥ Sequins.
- ♥ Rhinestones.
- ♥ Round rocaille beads.
- ♥ White pearls.
- ♥ Glitter.

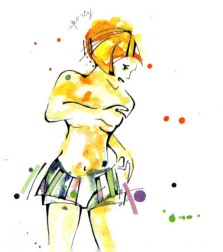
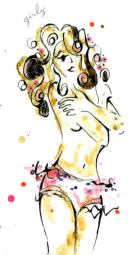

spicy suggestions

Wear your cestus out in public? Why not? Conceal your sparkling fancy pants under a skirt or a pair of jeans. If you have made a decorated scarf, toss it around your shoulders with pride! Strut your stuff as you walk tall down the street knowing that you are sporting a most magical pair of undies. It would be your secret as you pick up the morning newspaper, walk the dog, catch the bus for work, have an important meeting with your boss or client, or lunch with your friends. Others may wonder what is different about you, why you seem so confident, why the corners of your mouth are turned up in a half smile. You will know it is because you have found your inner Love Goddess and are starting to unleash her! Watch out, world!

If you want to let close girlfriends in on your secret, you can share with them the story of Aphrodite and her magical cestus. Hera, once a rival of Aphrodite for the title of "fairest" (Aphrodite won), even borrowed Aphrodite's magic girdle to recapture her husband's wayward love. Instead of letting your girlfriends borrow your magic undies, teach them how to create their own and infuse them with their own bewitching charms. This will make them irresistible to the hunk of their choosing. This Love Goddess stuff is so powerful that all potential Goddesses must agree to a code of ethics before unleashing their powers. This code states that whoever sees him first has first dibs. No stealing each other's hotties, please.

Wearing your cestus will give you confidence and a smile.

SPICY SUGGESTIONS 19

girl power

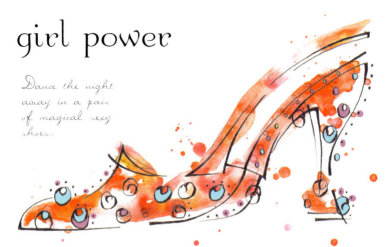

Dance the night away in a pair of magical, sexy shoes.

Perhaps fancy undies or glittering bras don't work for you. Maybe you are a bit more low-keyed or modest. Instead you can infuse your personal power into any object you choose. Think about how your favorite high heels make you feel as you strap them on for an evening of dancing. You stand taller and straighter. You walk with a swoosh as your hips sway in time with the click of your heels. Perhaps you have a favorite top that reveals just enough of your womanly charms. Putting it on makes you feel seductive with a hint of sassy playfulness. These are power items for you because they make you feel

Bold! Lusty! Brilliant! Witty! Gorgeous! when you wear them. It's almost like having a lucky charm in your pocket—you can do no wrong.

Get inspired to open wide the possibilities for power items! Do you have special earrings that you wear when you need to feel lucky? Is there a necklace that makes you feel especially alluring? What is it that you reach for when you need to feel confident?

A power object doesn't have to be something you wear. You can keep it in a special box and touch it for good luck. You can display it on your dressing-table. No one else has to know it is your power item—only you do.

These items are imbued with your own personal magic because you believe it to be so. Just as Aphrodite believed her magic cestus made her irresistible to men, you too can believe in the power of your fancy pants, your gilded T-shirt, your glittering bra, your red high heels, or your pearl earrings.

It's all up to you.

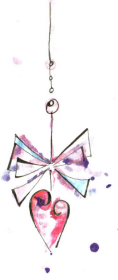

A pendant necklace can add fun and glamor.

taking it to the streets!

There are many places and ways to unleash your inner Goddess, some more appropriate than others. Please use discretion in public areas! Aphrodite's favorites are listed in the chapters to follow, but here are some other suggestions:

- ♥ Skinny-dipping after dark—keep that mosquito repellent handy.
- ♥ In the back row of the movie theater—a tried-and-true classic.
- ♥ In the first row of the roller coaster—Goddesses aren't afraid of anything!

Unleash your inner Goddess with a ride on a roller coaster.

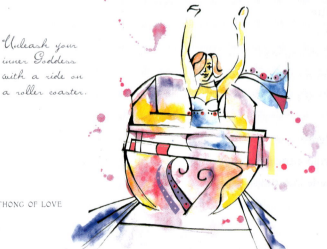

- ♥ On a long walk in the woods—the birds and the bees do it.
- ♥ At the back table of a restaurant—anyone for a game of footsie?
- ♥ Together on a motorcycle or moped if that's your speed—get all those parts vibrating.
- ♥ Knocking a seven ball in the corner pocket—watch his mouth drop when you pack your own stick to bring to the pool hall.
- ♥ Taking a carousel ride together—grab the golden rings from the side—and get another ride!
- ♥ Tent camping out in the woods—just you and your lover and . . . what was that noise?
- ♥ Attending an art opening or a museum event—impress him with your knowledge of surrealism.
- ♥ Ordering martinis in a hotel bar—all eyes are upon you.
- ♥ Have a couple's massage—so close, yet . . .

Remember, it's not what you do or where you go, it's your attitude! Get sexy, Goddess, and take that attitude into the streets!

LOVE NOTES

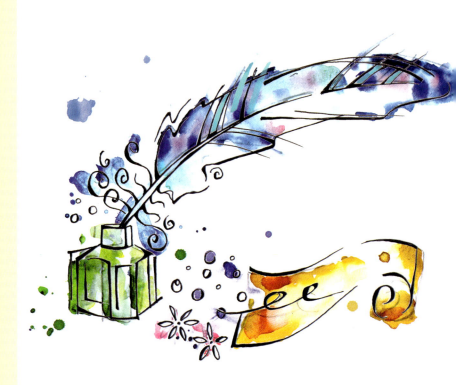

It is rumored that Aphrodite needed an entire room to hold all the love notes she received from her admirers. Aphrodite was the mistress of seductive conversation filled with gracious laughter, sweet musings, and the charms and delights of love. Her witty repartee kept admirers enthralled, waiting eagerly for her next delightful comment. When she could not see them in person, she kept them intrigued through her letter writing. Of course in those days there was really only one medium for love notes—papyrus, which was the ancient Greek version of paper. Today we have so many ways to let our lovers know how we feel about them.

As you prepare for an evening with your lover, you can set the tone by sending him messages through the day. Are you feeling Playful? Sassy? Shy? Erotic? Do you want the evening to be light and breezy, or are you looking for a serious commitment? Sometimes men need an extra push. Be bold, Goddess, and take the first step! Offer him something he cannot refuse—an evening of your undivided attention.

titillating technology

As your thoughts wander to getting down with your lover this evening, why not share some of those fantasies with him? You can use technology to get the evening off to a great start while you are both still at work or doing afternoon chores. Twenty-first century electronics is a great vehicle for getting someone's attention or for just connecting with your admirer. How wonderful it is to discover a message from your sweetie in your online mailbox! If Aphrodite were around today, she would probably be as addicted to her cell phone, e-mail, and Instant Message (IM) as the rest of us. Whereas she had to wait days for a hand-carried response via messenger, we can get results in minutes!

However, just because it is easy to send an e-mail or an IM doesn't mean you should overdo it. A Goddess chooses words that will titillate her admirer just enough to keep him hoping the next message is from her. Nobody likes a pest! Being mysterious is an incredible turn-on, even if you are showing your fun and playful side with goofy messages and silly icons.

Sending an e-mail is the modern-day version of dipping your feather quill into ink and writing a note to your man in flowery script. When you are feeling confident and Goddesslike, go ahead and send the first e-mail to a new admirer. He can take his own time to respond and is not put on the spot, as he would be if you phoned him. Many men still like to make the first move; sending a short e-mail gives them the encouragement and opportunity to make the first phone call.

E-mail messages can also be long and flowing and heartfelt, to be read over and over again. You should give as much thought to the contents of an e-mail—and whether or not to send it—as you would to a handwritten letter. Once you hit that "send" button, it cannot be retrieved. It goes without saying:

Go ahead and send a short e-mail to your sweetie.

be sure to check once, and then again, the name in the e-mail's "to" box. Too many electronic mails have been sent to the wrong person, with the sender never able to fully live down the incident, especially if the e-mail was sent to their boss or office mate instead of their lover!

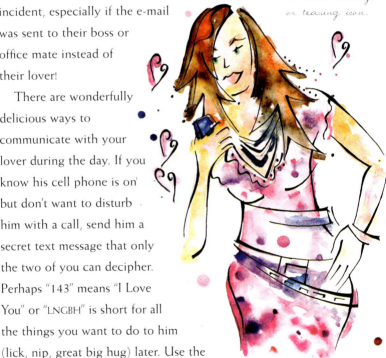

Stay connected by sending your love a secret message or teasing icon.

There are wonderfully delicious ways to communicate with your lover during the day. If you know his cell phone is on but don't want to disturb him with a call, send him a secret text message that only the two of you can decipher. Perhaps "143" means "I Love You" or "LNGBH" is short for all the things you want to do to him (lick, nip, great big hug) later. Use the photo feature to send a picture of yourself doing something naughty, or pose some stuffed animals if you are too modest. Perhaps photograph a street sign and send it to him as your rendezvous point for your evening activities.

Sending IMs are an easy way to stay connected. But be careful what you send via an IM, as people often walk away from their computer with IM still active, leaving your message available for any passerby to see. Or your lover might be showing his boss the latest financial projections when your IM pops up! Whoops!

It is often said that a picture is worth a thousand words, and technology offers its own style of pictures in the form of icons. Send your love a kissy face, or a big toothy grin, or perhaps flirtatious eyes. Icons come in all varieties, many of them animated for that extra punch. What better way to let your lover know you are thinking of him than by sending goofy icons throughout the day? The possibilities are as endless as your imagination.

Get creative and stand out from the crowd. Go, Cyber-Goddess!

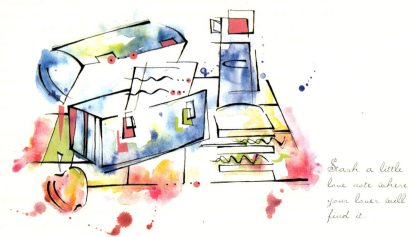

Stash a little love note where your lover will find it.

hidden notes

Leave little reminders of yourself around the house for your lover to find when you're not there. Think how he will feel when he reaches into his bathrobe pocket and pulls out an unexpected note from you! With every note he finds, his thoughts will return to times you've spent together. Choose just the right saying for the moment—"You're my hero!"; "Hi, Sexy, can't wait to spend another night with you!" Goddesses always know the right things to say to their man!

Here are some possible places to stash a little love note:

♥ In his underwear drawer, inside a pair of boxers.
♥ Taped to the bathroom mirror.
♥ Inside the case of his favorite CD.
♥ On his car's sun visor.
♥ In the suitcase he's taking on a business trip.
♥ In his lunch bag.
♥ Wrapped around his dog's collar.
♥ In his favorite pair of sneakers.
♥ In his gym bag.
♥ In the refrigerator taped to the carton of milk.
♥ Taped to the TV set.
♥ In his guitar case.
♥ Under his pillow.
♥ On the inside of his bedroom door.
♥ Sticky-noted on his computer monitor.
♥ In his favorite coffee mug.

Go wild, Love Goddess—the more unexpected the place, the bigger the surprise and the wider his smile!

go for broke!

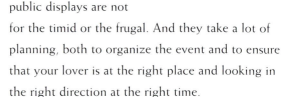

Sometimes nothing will do but a huge public declaration of your love. If you are sure he can handle it—and doubly sure he is worth it—then, go for broke! He will never forget it! Extreme public displays are not for the timid or the frugal. And they take a lot of planning, both to organize the event and to ensure that your lover is at the right place and looking in the right direction at the right time.

Perhaps you want to declare your feelings on the famous marquee in Times Square? The neon lights on Broadway are dazzling, but not as dazzling as you. (Would you happen to be wearing your magic cestus under that winter coat?) What about some skywriting as you and your man relax on your

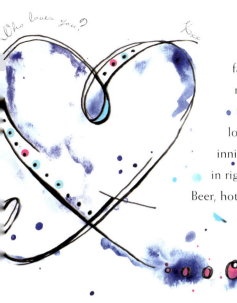

Who loves you?

favorite beach? A short message and calm skies are the trick to this extravagant love note. It's the seventh-inning stretch, and on the board in right field is your love message. Beer, hotdogs, and his name in lights are every man's dream of a perfect evening. Or how about a picnic in your favorite park as a trio of violinists serenade you and your man with your favorite love songs?

For lots of fun, consider a singing telegram. Have a personal message sung to your man by an actor in a gorilla suit or clown suit. Although public displays are not for everyone, on the right occasion these bold and dramatic messages surely say to your lover "You're worth it, and I want the world to know!"

GO FOR BROKE!

good old-fashioned class

For something completely different, why not catch him off guard with an old-fashioned perfumed letter written on fancy paper and sealed with a wax heart? The mailman will wonder what your man did to deserve such personal attention. An unsuspecting neighbor might wonder why her bills, carried in the same mail pouch, smell so good!

Take yourself shopping to a marvelous stationery store. Browse through the writing papers—bark paper, rice paper, marbled stationery crafted in Florence, Italy, 100 percent cotton sheets. Touch the rich textures, let your eyes take in the vibrant colors. Peruse the pens. A letter crafted with an old-fashioned fountain pen has a unique charm. Check out the wax seals and colored sealing waxes, which can add that personal touch. Picture yourself writing the most enchanting love letter you can conjure with a beautiful burgundy fountain pen, slipping the folded letter into its envelope, then lighting a stick of sealing wax and watching the wax slowly and sensuously drip onto the back of your envelope. While the wax is warm, lovingly press into it the seal of a heart or dove or perhaps the first initial of your name, knowing that only your lover will break the seal. Finally, mist the envelope with your favorite fragrance. Steamy!

This elegant endeavor demonstrates that you are both a Goddess of Romance and a Goddess of Class. The name on the front of that envelope belongs to one very lucky guy.

Your favorite fragrance will add a finishing touch to your note.

A BATH OF ROSE PETALS

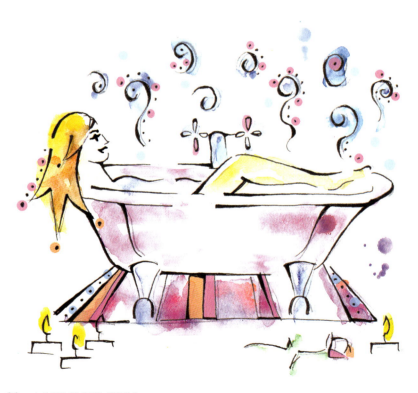

Strip off those ordinary clothes. Light some candles. Step into a warm bath filled with rose petals. When was the last time you really pampered yourself and let your Love Goddess out?

The rose has long been the symbol of love and passion. The ancient Greeks strewed rose petals before kings and queens marching in processions. Poets have written sonnets to their mistresses' rosy cheeks. Even the great Cleopatra used to perfume herself with rose oil before an evening with Mark Antony. Adonis loved to surprise Aphrodite as she bathed in her favorite mountain spring, which was laced with freshly picked rose petals. The sun would set and the moon would rise high in the sky before the two of them gave even a thought to ending their "bath." Every Love Goddess should have a vase of roses in her bedroom or a bottle of rose oil handy, as the fragrance evokes feelings of passion and love.

Roses best reveal their magic when their petals meet with warm water, releasing the rose's essential oils. Discover what special mysteries the rose holds for you.

bare essentials

- ♥ Get about a dozen roses. You can use wild roses, long-stemmed roses, or roses from your backyard. It's fine to combine roses of many colors, as each color adds a different essence of love to your bath water. Red conveys passion and respect. Pink signifies happiness, admiration, and friendship. White suggests spiritual love and purity. Yellow roses stand for friendship, joy, and gladness. Lavender symbolizes enchantment and love at first sight.
- ♥ Collect lots of candles. You may want to set a mood by using just red tapers or go wild with candles of many colors and shapes. Variety is the spice of life for any Love Goddess!

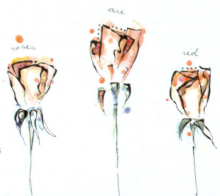

roses are red

- ♥ Over-sized fluffy towels feel so good against the skin. Splurge and buy some bright red towels to heighten passion or perhaps lavender ones to provoke enchantment. Pile up plenty.
- ♥ Set out a pitcher to pour water over your body when you are in the bath.
- ♥ Choose music and set up the CD player. What music puts you in the mood for love? Smoky jazz? Puccini arias? Indian flutes and drums? Maybe try something new for this special night.
- ♥ This is your time to relax. So go ahead and fantasize about the evening ahead with your lover as you collect your bath essentials. Nobody else needs to know what you are thinking about.

Have your towel and pitcher handy for when you are in your bath.

BARE ESSENTIALS

it's bath time, goddess!

- ♥ Set the mood by turning down the lights in other rooms.
- ♥ If it is wintertime, turn up the heat or light a fire in the fireplace.
- ♥ Candlelight is very flattering. Surround yourself with it, placing candles along the way from your bedroom to your bathroom and in various places around your bathtub.
- ♥ Fill the tub with deliciously warm water.
- ♥ All Love Goddesses have a sexy robe. You may feel sexiest in your boyfriend's football jersey or a flannel shirt or a hand-embroidered long silk robe. Whatever it is, put it on and follow the candlelit path to your bath. Walk tall! Be proud! You are a Love Goddess!
- ♥ Take a handful of roses and crush the petals as you drop them into the bath water. Rose petals are sexy. Rose petals and attitude are sexier!
- ♥ As you drop the petals into the water, and before you step in, get in touch with your Love Goddess using these words or words of your own:

I am one sexy Love Goddess!
My powers of seduction know no limits.
I ask for what I need and get exactly what I want.
Tonight is MY night.

- ♥ Yow! Slip into the bath waters and relax as the soft petals tickle your skin.
- ♥ Inhale the fragrance of roses. Feel their magical powers infusing you with allure and confidence. Imagine each color you have selected filling you with its own unique power. Passion! Happiness! Purity! Joy! Enhancement!
- ♥ Scoop up water with your pitcher and pour it over your arms, your legs, your back, your chest, and your head. Shower yourself with rose power!
- ♥ Aphrodite loved to bathe in mountain springs. Her admirers, of which she had many, would often hide among the bushes, hoping to catch a glimpse of her soft, luxurious body. She would

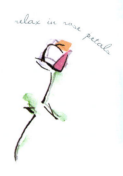

relax in rose petals

tease them as she washed herself, exposing first her leg, then perhaps her breast. Think of all the ways that you can tease your lover as the hours unfold. A seductive phone message, a sideways look, the bare curve of your back peeking out as you bend forward to get something out of the refrigerator for dinner. Follow Aphrodite's lead and bring back the lost art of the tease.

♥ Lie back in the bath and close your eyes. Imagine that you are with your man. Light up your mental movie screen and let it show you some of things you might do together. Start with your favorite scenes and then add some new twists. No holds barred, Love Goddess!

♥ As you prepare to step out of your bath, take a deep breath and remember how you are feeling right now. Let the rose petals swirl around you as you reach for that fluffy towel and dry off. Don't worry if a few petals cling to your skin; your lover will be sure to find them later . . .

♥ You are confident, powerful, and sexy! You'll know *exactly* what to do when your lover arrives.

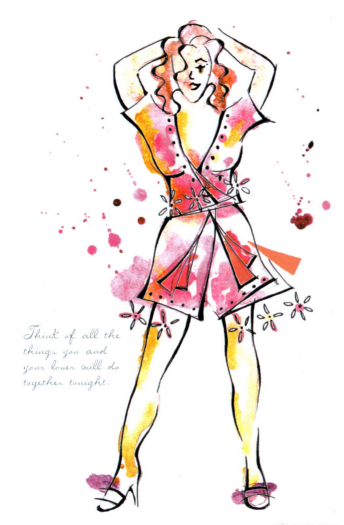

Think of all the things you and your lover will do together tonight.

IT'S BATH TIME, GODDESS!

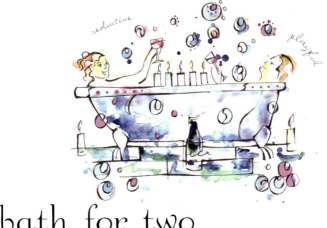

bath for two

Is it better to give or receive? When it comes to bath time with your lover, the answer is—yes! Bathing together is a wonderful way to explore each other's bodies, finding all those ticklish spots and trying out your new massage techniques. Bath time can be silly and fun or it can be steamy and seductive or a bit of both. Decide what kind of mood you want to create and let the games begin!

Splash down!

Aphrodite loved the bubbles that formed where the waterfall at the edge of her bathing grotto met the mountain spring. You can recreate that effect by filling your tub with a bubble bath. For a bit of fun, gather a rubber ducky or two, some water pistols and bath paint if you are feeling particularly adventuresome. Have fun hiding underneath the bubbles, surprise-attacking each other with water pistols, or concocting elaborate stories about life on a desert island with just a rubber ducky for company. With the bath paints, paint each other in the style of your favorite cartoon character. Laughter is sexy.

Steam up those windows!

Sometimes the day demands a luxurious and arousing bathing experience at its end. Play the aggressor as you let your lover rest against you. Reach around his body and begin to wash his hands. Spend time with each of his fingers, savoring their shape. See how the silky water slides off his arm. Feel the power throbbing within them as you imagine his arms encircling you later. Whew! This Love Goddess stuff can get really hot! Now you know why Aphrodite and Adonis lost track of time, enthralled with their day-into-night bathing adventures.

What a delicious way to start the evening!

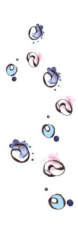

sense-sation

Aphrodite combined sensations from all the senses when she wanted to create an enthralling evening. Even the ultimate Love Goddess knows that looks aren't enough, even if she is ravishing! As you plan each part of your evening, remember to satisfy each sensory need. Capturing your lover's sense of sight is easy—how could he possibly take his eyes off you! The elements of water and skin-against-skin in your rose petal bath provide a tingling introduction to the sense of touch. What could be more musical to his ears than the sound of your voice? Try speaking softly to draw him closer.

After the bath, your body will be positively glowing with the delicious scent of roses. To keep him hovering close by, try a few drops of rose water or essential oil of rose diluted in a carrier oil, such as almond, in those secret spots. Fragrances have an uncanny power to move us. A whiff of freshly baked bread, a particular flower, or a long-forgotten scent can instantly conjure up scenes and emotions from the past. Use this potent yet often-overlooked faculty to ensure that your lover remembers you long after you have moved on. Every time he smells roses he will recall the evening of enchantment he spent in your presence.

The sense of taste is closely connected to the sense of smell. The old folk saying, "The way to a man's heart is through his stomach," may have more to do with smell than with taste. Read on to enter a realm of aroma and flavor, texture and presentation, as they combine to create a delectable and unforgettable meal.

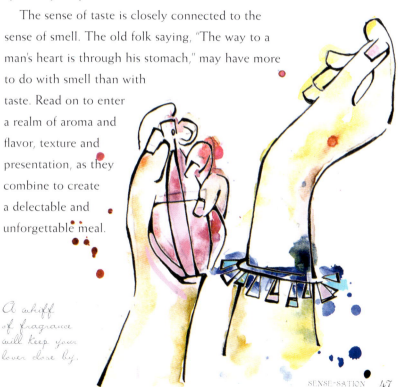

A whiff of fragrance will keep your lover close by.

DINNER DELIGHTS

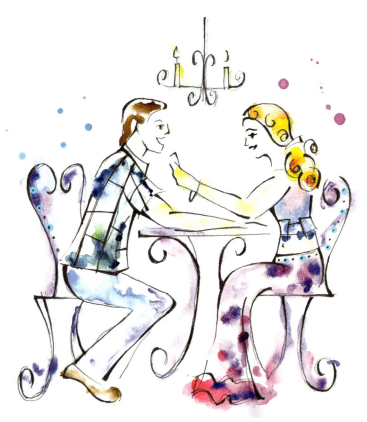

Food fuels not only the body but also the soul. To prepare a meal for someone you love is like offering them a part of yourself. Stories recount that Aphrodite could make men cry, laugh, fall in love, and howl at the moon just by eating food she had prepared. Now that's some kind of cook!

Know that you can infuse your meals with whatever qualities you choose. So think lusty thoughts as you prepare the meal and you will be sure to have your lover eating out of your hand. In fact, Aphrodite felt that utensils only got in the way. Those sharp knives and forks could hurt someone! Instead, focus on the sense of touch as you feed your lover by hand and he in turn does the same for you.

planning and shopping

One of Aphrodite's favorite meals to bewitch a man consists of:

- ♥ Wickedly good rustic bread dipped in olive oil.
- ♥ Scrumptious whole black and green olives (yes, with the pits still in).
- ♥ Luscious raw oysters on the half shell.
- ♥ Ambrosial sautéed shrimp and garlic in oil over spaghetti.
- ♥ Delectable sautéed mushrooms in butter.
- ♥ Exquisite red or white wine.

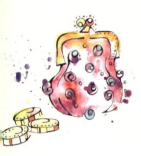

When you go shopping buy the best and freshest ingredients.

Plan to shop the same day for the shrimp and oysters. Everything else can be purchased ahead. Locate a neighborhood gourmet store, wine shop, and a store that sells good fresh fish. Buy the shrimp peeled and deveined and the oysters already opened. There are some things a Love Goddess should just never have to do! Select a whole loaf of unsliced bread, an assortment of olives, and your favorite mushrooms from the gourmet store. If the shop has prepared sautéed mushrooms that you can just take home and heat up, even better! Buy a good quality pasta. Ask the wine seller for suggestions on either red or white wine. Tell him what you are serving so he can match the wine to the food.

Your shopping bags should be full of all sorts of sensuous delicacies..

Of course, make sure that your lover is not allergic to anything on your menu. Shellfish can be particularly troublesome for some people. Substitute any of the above suggestions with food of your own choosing.

Be sure to consider how it will complement the other items you are serving. Since this is a hand-to-mouth experience, choose food that does not have to be cut into pieces to be eaten. It's more fun if the food you pick is drippy, slippery, and sloppy! What man can resist licking a stream of warm oil sliding down a Goddess's chin? After all, he is only mortal!

meal preparation

- ♥ Give yourself plenty of time to prepare the meal, especially if it is food you have never made before. Look to your favorite cookbooks or your mother (if you love her cooking) for specific instructions and preparation tips.
- ♥ Boil a pot of water on the stove for the spaghetti.
- ♥ Arrange the oysters on a serving platter. Cut up some lemon slices and arrange them alongside the oysters. Cover the platter and put it in the refrigerator to keep cool.
- ♥ Drain the liquid from the olives and put them in a bowl. They can remain at room temperature.
- ♥ Cut up the mushrooms and sauté them in butter. Then put them in an ovenproof bowl and pop them into a warm oven until ready to serve.
- ♥ Sauté the shrimp in garlic and oil until cooked. Remove the shrimp.
- ♥ Put spaghetti in the boiling water and cook until done.
- ♥ Drain the spaghetti and add it to the pan with garlic and oil. Sauté lightly.

- ♥ Toss the shrimp with the spaghetti, garlic, and oil, and transfer to a serving bowl. Put it in the oven to keep warm.
- ♥ Tear the bread into large chunks and put the pieces in a serving bowl. Pour olive oil into a small bowl for dipping.
- ♥ Think erotic thoughts as you slice the mushrooms and toss the spaghetti. Inhale the smells of freshly sautéed garlic and shrimp simmering in oil. Mmmmmmmm. Yummy! Picture your lover as he nibbles on an olive you are holding in your fingers. Mmmmmmm, even yummier!
- ♥ Have fun cooking!
- ♥ Open the wine. Why not pour a glass for yourself?

Congratulations on cooking up a heavenly meal. Aphrodite would be proud! It's time to set out plates, wine glasses, and napkins. No utensils, please!

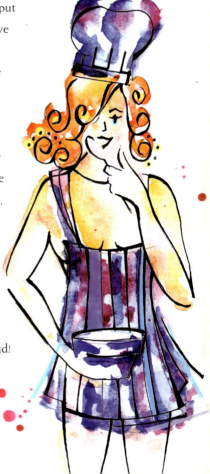

Think erotic thoughts as you prepare the meal.

arranging the space

Aphrodite felt too much of life is spent sitting and standing and not enough lying down and relaxing. One could always find her stretched out in a chaise lounge (although they didn't call them chaise lounges back then) with admiring men at her feet offering to satisfy her every desire. The environment in which you offer food and drink to your lover is as important as what you are serving. Consider the difference between sitting on plastic chairs at a plastic table in a fast-food restaurant and reclining on a blanket at the beach watching the sunset. As a Love Goddess, you need to hold a higher standard than the general public. Therefore

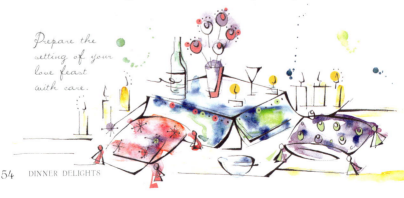

Prepare the setting of your love feast with care.

take your time to decide where to situate your love feast and how the space should be arranged.

Perhaps you can set up a bunch of cozy pillows on a blanket in front of the fireplace. Maybe you can push the dining table into a corner and spread a tablecloth in the middle of the dining room floor. Your cocktail table could be the perfect height on which to arrange your bewitching display of taste delights as you and your lover sit on the floor next to it. Or you might want to take the feast outside. Two chaise lounges set head-to-toe next to each other might be just the thing. Or an intimate table for two on the patio or in a secluded part of the garden could provide privacy and connection with nature.

Be creative, go wild! You know how to create the perfect setting for your lover. Think: pillows; a comfortable place to sit; candles and soft lighting; intoxicating music; a blanket, sheet, or tablecloth on which to spread out your feast. Shut off the ringer on your phone, and hang a Do Not Disturb sign on the door!

naughty nibbles

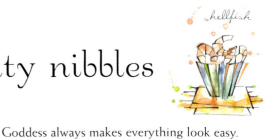

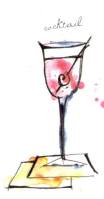

A Goddess always makes everything look easy. Make sure you allow enough time after cooking to change into your evening attire. Remember to wear one of your power items! Light the candles where you will be dining, turn on the music, and check on the food. When your lover rings the doorbell, you should be relaxing with a glass of wine or a cocktail in hand looking like the ultimate Naughty Nibbles Goddess. He may want to begin devouring you right away. Aphrodite often had to put her suitors into a trance to give herself a rest. You might just suggest that it will be a long evening and wouldn't it be more fun to go slowly? Pour him a glass of wine or his favorite cocktail.

When you are ready to begin enjoying your scrumptious feast, invite your lover into the space you have created. Have him close his eyes so his other senses become more acute. Bring in the bowl of bread chunks with the olive oil for dipping, the olives, the platter of raw oysters, the bowl of spaghetti and shrimp sautéed in garlic and oil, and the mushrooms in butter. Tuck a napkin under his chin. Ask him to describe what he smells. Hold each platter or bowl under his nose and see if he can guess what it contains. Feed him a little of each food offering with your fingers until his mind is swirling with smells, textures, and tastes. This is no ordinary dinner date!

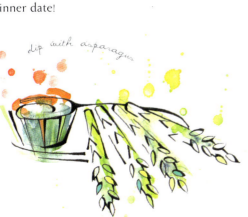

olives

dip with asparagus

licking fingers

Time to dig into your prepared feast. Use fingers only!

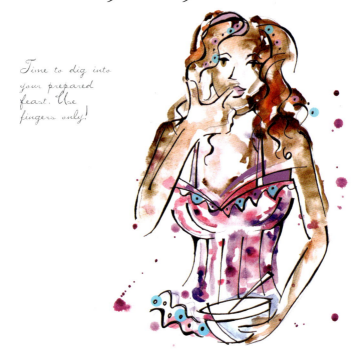

Now that you have completely tormented your lover as only a Goddess could do, it's time to dig in to the feast. If your lover is wondering where the utensils are, tell him there are none and he will have to be creative. Not many restaurants would tolerate the behavior you two are about to exhibit.

Start with something simple, like feeding him an olive. Next, dip some bread into the oil and hold it up to your lover's mouth. No one says you can't accidentally miss and get oil on the tip of his nose! Guess you'll just have to lick it off. Oysters are wondrously slippery and fun to eat as they slide off their shells into your mouth. Try holding one with your fingers and feeding it to your lover. Oysters are said to be an aphrodisiac, which means they arouse sexual desires. Of course, being a protégée of Aphrodite, pretty much anything you do is an aphrodisiac! Are you feeling confident enough to serve spaghetti to each other? Who knew spaghetti in oil could feel so good in your hands? Don't forget the shrimp! And those buttery mushrooms are still waiting to be devoured. Hands, fingers, mouths, elbows, feet (sure, why not?) are all valid utensils for this meal. Make sure your lover feeds you in return.

Washing the dishes can wait until morning . . .

THE DANCE OF THE VEILS

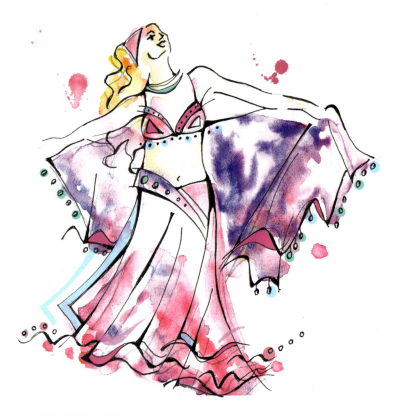

Legend tells us that as Aphrodite prepared to dance for one of her suitors, her friends the Graces would anoint her body with fragrant oils and adorn her with her most precious jewels. When she danced, it is said, her veil was more dazzling than flame and her delicate bosom shone like the moon.

Woman have been dancing with veils for centuries. On the island of Cyprus, mysteries were celebrated honoring Aphrodite as the goddess of human love and fertility. Ecstatic and lewd dances using the tympanum, a type of cymbal, were a feature of these rites. You can join the ranks of women from ancient Greece, India, Persia, Egypt, and Turkey to many countries today who have dared to lower the veil and shake and shimmy for their men. You can dance the dance of love, lust or beauty, or even the dance of sheer joy or laughter.

Somewhere far back in your family history, maybe a far-distant relative enticed her suitor into marriage through a mysterious and captivating veil dance. Who knows? What kind of effect do you want to have on your man tonight?

preparation

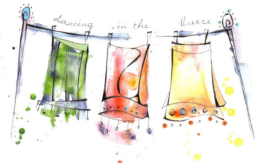

Veils come in all shapes and sizes. You might already have a beautiful piece of fabric—perhaps a scarf. The best fabric is sheer or semisheer. It should also be lightweight so it floats gracefully behind you and is easy to swish! Silk, chiffon, and polyester make good veils. The ideal shape is rectangular—wide enough for you to hold with arms stretched wide over your head with some extra fabric dangling on each side. Shop around to find exotic materials suitable for a veil. You could type the words "belly dance veil" into any on-line search engine for a selection of companies that sell them. Of course, you can also purchase some wonderful material at your neighborhood fabric store. Pick a color from their range that makes you feel very, very sexy.

Plan to have a large enough area to perform your dance. Make sure there are no overhead fixtures that the veil can get caught on or lit candles that can ignite your veil. Your man also needs a comfortable place to sit so he can enjoy watching you. Perhaps the space where you enjoyed dinner is appropriate. Or maybe it's time to move into the bedroom.

Within the wide selection of music available is something to suit any evening's mood. Traditional belly dance music typically consists of complex and unusual rhythm patterns. Look in the world music section of your record store under "belly dance" or "Middle East" for compilation CDs that will give you a good idea of the different types of traditional music. On the other hand, nobody says that you can't dance to your favorite artists. What about some hip-grinding Latin? Or some slow and sexy rhythm and blues? Or even some head-banging rock 'n' roll? You're the Goddess. You decide.

dance with the veil

When people want to celebrate, they dance! Tonight, Goddess, is a celebration of your feminine power. So give it all you have! Of course you will want to wear your cestus, scarf, or power item for that extra bit of magic in your step. Let's sizzle!

There are few things sexier than the sight of a scantily clad Goddess strolling seductively into a room behind a sheer veil to pulsating music. Dancing and swishing with abandon may look complicated, but it is really quite easy.

Get used to the veil by stretching out your arms and holding it tightly but comfortably between each thumb and index finger or each index and middle finger. Move around the room, keeping the veil fluttering behind you by lifting your arms up and down. Bring the veil below your eyes to hide all but your eyes mysteriously behind it. Now flip it over your head in a circular motion, arms held high, and let it flutter behind you as you walk. Lower your arms to hip height and drag the veil behind you. Play with sweeping it in circles over your head and in circles on each side of your body. Spiral yourself in your veil and then slowly unwind to reveal yourself in all your beauty. Let yourself go to the sound and rhythm of the music. Move your body in ways that feel right to you. Let the veil dance you!

Set free your sensuous Goddess force when you dance with the veil.

If you like, you can use your veil in combination with the traditional hypnotic undulations and hip movements that characterize the ancient art of belly dancing. Dancing in this way sets free the sensuous, passionate Goddess force that is lurking just underneath your business clothes, waiting for the opportunity to escape.

Experiment with moving your hips in a small circle, then move your feet farther apart and rotate your hips in a large circle. Rock your hips forward and back and then side to side. With your feet apart, use your hips to trace the shape of a figure eight parallel to the floor. Arm poses can be very dramatic. Hold your palms together over your head as if in prayer. Your veil can trail behind your body. Try moving your arms in a snakelike fashion both in front of your body and at your sides. Shimmy the upper half of your body and then the lower half. Can you shimmy everything at once? Play with the movements. Think about smooth, flowing, complex, and sensual moves, alternated with shaking and shimmying ones.

Your eyes are a primary element of the dance. When you cover your body and only your eyes show, all attention is drawn to them. In traditional dances, the dancer might acknowledge her audience with occasional glances or brief little smiles. But in veil dancing she draws her audience in with her eyes. Direct your eyes to the part of your body where you want your man to look. If you are rotating your hips, cast your eyes in that direction, and he will tend to look there also. If you focus on the sensuous movements of your arms, so will he.

You may want to begin your dance from a position on the floor, swirling your veil around as you emerge, as if from a cocoon. Or you can start in a standing position and finish on your knees as the music slows down.

Practice veil dancing to the music before your big evening together. Anything goes. Your lover is sure to be in awe of your grace and aroused by your moves. Have a blast, Goddess. Let loose and dance.

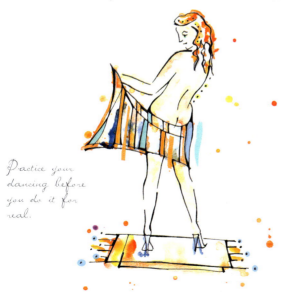

Practice your dancing before you do it for real.

striptease

In a striptease dance, the goal is to "tease" your audience by very slowly and provocatively removing each article of your clothing. The game is in the getting there. And everyone's a winner in this game!

Decide which clothes you want to wear as you make your entrance. A simple T-shirt and jeans or a suit jacket and skirt can be deceivingly suggestive. It's all in the attitude. Be sure to wear your magic cestus underneath, as you'll want to reveal that last. Select music that really lights your fire like some thumping reggae or perhaps something classical like Ravel's *Bolero*.

The classic striptease has always started with the dancer deliberating removing her full-length gloves finger by finger. Can't you just imagine the men in the audience thinking "Hurry up, hurry up!" yet enjoying every delicious minute of the dance? Since gloves are not a typical wardrobe item for

slinky undergarments

today's Goddess, start with something simple, like removing your shoes or letting loose your hair.

As you continue to seductively remove your clothing, or hint at removing your clothing by showing a bra strap or the band of your thong undies, keep your body in motion. An inviting hip undulation or a backwards look over your shoulder will keep him screaming for more, more, more! Have fun with the tease. Make it up as you go along. You can do no wrong, Goddess! Ooo la la!

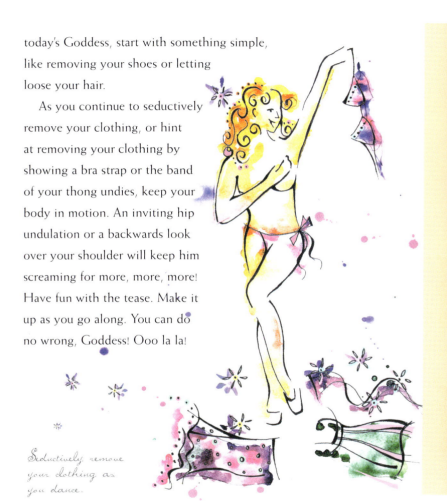

Seductively remove your clothing as you dance.

shadow dancing

For an unusual treat, entertain your lover by taking center stage in your own shadow dance. To picture the set-up for this dance, imagine a life-size version of a puppet theater, where the puppet characters appear behind a backlit opaque screen. All that the audience can see is their silhouettes. Very mysterious!

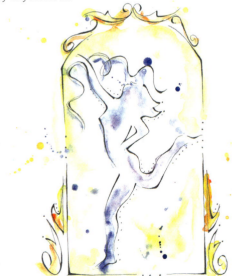

Entertain your lover with a mysterious shadow dance.

To set the stage for your performance, hang a sheet over a doorway so it covers the opening entirely. Then arrange the lighting behind the sheet so a clear silhouette falls on your screen when you stand directly behind it. The room where your lover will sit should be fairly dark, so all his attention is drawn to your shadow on the screen. Your selection of music should match the mood you want to create.

Start your dance fully clothed. Maybe you want just the shadow of a leg or an arm to fall on the screen before you move your entire silhouette into view. You can move in and out of sight, playing a little game of hide and seek. Taking off your clothes behind the screen is wildly exciting, as your lover can see the outline of your ravishing curves, but nothing more. If you are feeling particularly erotic, use the security of the screen to do things you might be too shy to do in person. He will surely be totally mad for you by the time you reveal yourself in the flesh.

This is a hot one, Goddess. Use with extreme caution. Maybe you should have a bucket of water handy in case your man gets too steamed up!

BODY PAINTING DESSERT

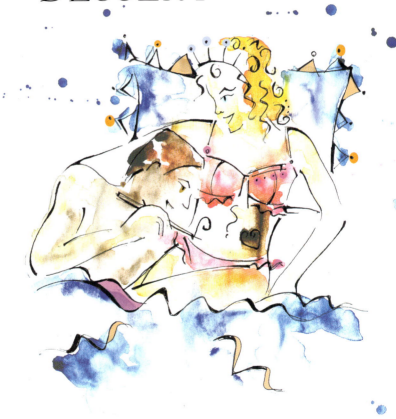

Remember how much you loved to finger paint as a kid? It was one of the few times you were allowed to get messy and your parents didn't yell at you. Body painting with food is the adult version of finger painting, except much, much better. In this version, you get to eat your creations! This feast can get a bit sticky, but that is part of the fun.

After all that dancing, you and your lover are bound to be hungry. Adonis was fond of feeding grapes and other delicacies to Aphrodite as she reclined in her favorite lounge chair. You can take this a few steps further by using your body as a platter and offering yourself as dessert to your lover. Let your man decorate your body with his favorite desserts and then dig in! Yummy! Now switch positions and return the favor. Double yummy!

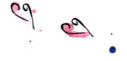

desserts to devour

Choose desserts that are sweet and spreadable and easy to prepare. When you are out shopping for dinner, pick up some of your favorite dessert items. Here are some of Aphrodite's suggestions:

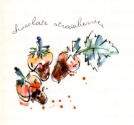
chocolate strawberries

- ♥ Heavy cream with just a touch of sugar. Whip up your own into a smooth mass of creamy peaks, or cheat (Goddesses never really cheat, they just have more important things to do with their time!) by buying a can of whipped cream.
- ♥ Buy the best dark chocolate you can afford. Melt it in a double boiler to create chocolate ambrosia. Make sure it is cooled down sufficiently before you use it—you wouldn't want to burn any sensitive areas! Or cheat (that is, prioritize your time) by buying chocolate syrup and heating it up.
- ♥ Who can resist strawberries for dessert? Dip in melted chocolate or buy a basket of fresh berries

and purée them in a blender with a little sugar. If they are not in season, buy a bag of frozen strawberries or any other berry of your liking and purée to a luscious consistency.

Make a dessert that is sweet to savor and simple to spread.

♥ How about some honey for your honey? There are many varieties of honey to pick from. Select one that has a squeezable container for easy dripping.

♥ Maybe some applesauce would be fun! Choose some mixed with blackberry or cherry for a striking color.

♥ Jam makes wonderful body paint. Go for your favorite color or flavor.

♥ What about some peanut butter? Use the creamy kind.

♥ If you really want to get messy, cook up some chocolate pudding. It goes well with the whipped cream.

♥ And if you want to spend the night chasing your dessert, try some jello. Getting it to sit still on your man's body will certainly be entertaining!

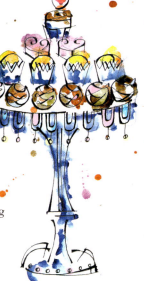

evocative designs

Now that you have all these delectable goodies to choose from, what are you going to draw on your lover's body? One approach is to cover him with evocative designs. Think of symbols or images that evoke strong feelings in you or are meaningful for both you and him.

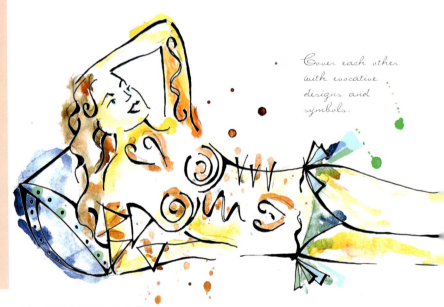

Cover each other with evocative designs and symbols.

Maybe you want to cover his whole body with chocolate spirals. How about a puréed strawberry snake slithering up his thigh? Or a whipped cream crescent moon on his forehead? A downward pointing triangle is an ancient Goddess symbol. You might draw the outline in chocolate syrup and fill in the center with raspberry jam. Simply delectable!

You could represent the gender symbols in honey. Maybe add some chocolate sprinkles on top! These symbols are astrological signs handed down from ancient Roman times. The pointed male symbol is the sign for Mars, and the female symbol with the cross represents Venus. How about a peace symbol outlined in whipped cream?

A yin-yang figure would be particularly striking—and delicious—in peanut butter and jelly. Who needs the bread! Get silly. Draw a happy face with chocolate pudding. For color, add some green jello pieces for eyes!

Go creative and cover your bodies from head to toe. The more you put on, the more you'll have to lick off later! Yow!

look at you!

Aphrodite was also known as the Goddess of Laughter. Laughter is a marvelous aphrodisiac. Besides being fun, laughing releases muscle tension, which is a wonderful precursor to "pillow talk." Aphrodite knew that gentle humor was just the right remedy when her man was upset about something or was feeling a little uncomfortable. Laughter makes us relax, and before we know it we have forgotten what we were upset about. Aphrodite was one smart cookie.

So when you see your sweetheart covered from head to toe in chocolate spirals, let loose with some peals and yucks. Or maybe shy giggles or a snort or two are more your style. Show him you are not afraid to look silly and have a good time. Laughter is joyous and infectious. Have you ever noticed that kids laugh far more than adults do? Be a kid again tonight and get the giggles until tears are streaming down your face. Not only does laughing puts a sexy twinkle in your eye that your man will find

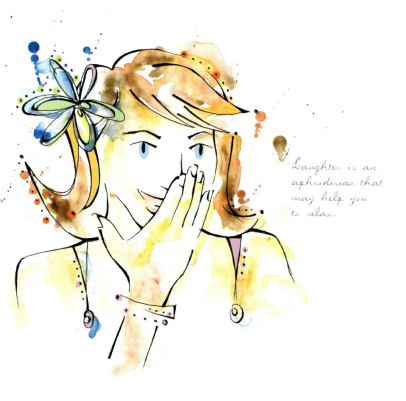

Laughter is an aphrodisiac that may help you to relax.

irresistible, but you will also develop abdominal muscles of steel from all those belly contractions!

It takes a courageous woman to laugh at herself and at life. You've got what it takes, Goddess! Go ahead, let go and have a blast!

animal pleasures

Are you feeling particularly animalistic tonight? There's nothing wrong with a little play-acting as long as no one gets hurt. We are all physical human beings, and sometimes the animal in us is just roaring to get out! So have some fun with your dessert feast and paint each other into the animal that is lurking just beneath the surface.

Bring out the wildness in both of you by painting tiger stripes or leopard spots on each other. Perhaps you have always wanted to be a wolf or a bear, a wild stallion or a wise old hoot owl. Indulge your fantasies! Create the plumage of a peacock on your man and let him strut his stuff! Are you feeling a bit feline this evening? Bring out your stealthy grace by having your man turn you into your favorite kitty. Meow! Is *101 Dalmatians* your all-time favorite movie? Turn each other into the cutest little pups ever seen this side of a Hollywood back lot.

Perhaps snakes are more your style. The serpent is worshipped in many cultures for its wisdom and magical powers. Paint each other with multicolored bands, bright speckles, and glorious patterns. Do you feel graceful and sensual? Charm each other with your serpentine ways.

Do your tastes run more to mythical creatures? Have you always wanted to be a mermaid or a dragon or a sphinx? Now is your chance to embody the attributes of these creatures. Paint yourself into mythology. Do you feel different?

Bring out the tiger or pussy cat in you by indulging in your fantasies.

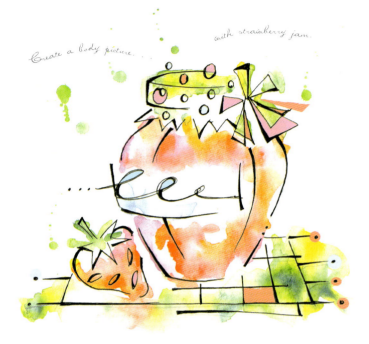

Create a body picture... with strawberry jam.

do it!

G o ahead and do it! Paint each other's bodies! Dance! Laugh! Become that tiger or that mermaid or one giant happy face, if only for one evening. If you don't like what you have drawn, lick it off and start again! The fun is in creating, in letting your spirits soar high, in being able to laugh with each other and at yourself, in feeling completely free with your partner to experiment, and letting yourself be wickedly lustful or softly erotic.

Your body is the perfect canvas. It is nonporous and completely washable! What better way to get to know each other than to offer up your bodies for art? So dip your finger into some chocolate and start drawing. Shake up that can of whipped cream and paint a picture. Dribble on some strawberry jam. Put your modesty in the closet for an evening and get down to business. Soon you will be so caught up in the silliness of the act that you won't care how you look.

The best part is cleaning up. Attack your favorite foods first. Or maybe start with the part of his body of which you are most fond. Maybe begin by licking off all the chocolate, then move on to the whipped cream, then the jelly. Be careful not to drool too much! This will surely be a dessert to remember.

Now when you call your lover a real "dish," it takes on a whole new meaning.

PILLOW TALK

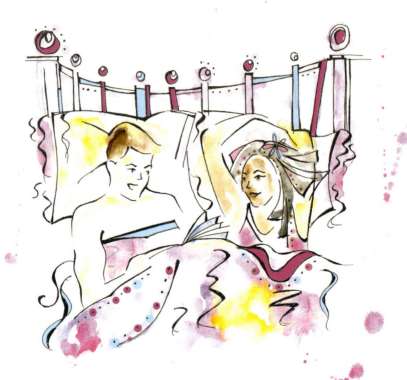

As evening turns into night, and the world begins to hush, it is time to reflect upon your most incredible evening (did you really do all those things?) and express your appreciation and love for each other. Poetry has been described as the voice of the angels, the sweet nectar of life. What is it about poetry that so deeply touches our souls?

A poem is a gift to be treasured. A poem continues to inspire us with new meanings every time as we read and reread it. Poets see the world differently. Their words are eternal—as true today as the day they were written.

You may never have considered poetry as something that would interest you. Maybe you were forced to read it in school and hated it because no one took the time to bring it to life for you. But the great poets, especially the love poets of today as well as ages past, are masters at deciphering the human condition and putting into words those feelings that so many of us share but are afraid to voice. You can freely express your love for your man using the words that the poets wrote just for that purpose.

poetry of love

Have you ever read a love poem by one of the classic love poets? Have you ever read one out loud to someone you love? Reading a poem out loud creates a special atmosphere. The words come alive. Take the opportunity tonight to select a few poems and read them to your lover. Here are some suggestions for love poetry to spice up your night and put words to your feelings. These selections can be found at the library or your local bookstore as well as on the Internet. But don't be limited by these. Go searching for the poems that will be your favorites.

Select a favorite poem to read to your lover.

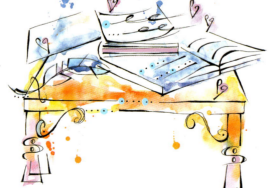

- ♥ "How Do I Love Thee?" by Elizabeth Barrett Browning.
- ♥ "Shall I Compare Thee to a Summer's Day?" by William Shakespeare.
- ♥ "Choice" by Angela Morgan.
- ♥ "Give All to Love" by Ralph Waldo Emerson.
- ♥ "The Passionate Shepard to His Love" by Christopher Marlowe.
- ♥ "The Owl and the Pussycat" by Edward Lear.
- ♥ "Love's Philosophy" by Percy Bysshe Shelley.
- ♥ "It Is Marvelous to Wake Up Together" by Elizabeth Bishop.
- ♥ "The Night the Children Were Away" by Stephen Dunn.
- ♥ "After Making Love We Hear Footsteps" by Galway Kinnell.
- ♥ "For What Binds Us" by Jane Hirshfield.
- ♥ "I Could Take" by Hayden Carruth.
- ♥ "Love Sonnet XI" by Pablo Neruda.
- ♥ "Day That I Have Loved" by Rubert Brooke.
- ♥ "To the Evening Star" by William Blake.

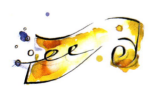

preparing the space

Reading poetry to each other is special no matter where you do it—in the woods, driving together in the car, at the beach—but it takes on extra meaning when you are lying cuddled in each other's arms in the privacy of your bedroom. Of all the places in your home, your bedroom best reflects your uniqueness, as it is your own personal space. Inviting a man into that space means you trust him and want to share that special part of you with him. You don't think Aphrodite let just anyone into her boudoir, do you?

To set the right atmosphere, consider all the senses. Place lots of candles around the room, or put your lamps on dimmers. For a really exotic look, you may even want to replace some of your regular light bulbs with colored ones. Pick one, or a few, essential oils—the ones you are drawn to are the right ones for the evening. Lavender is a wonderful calming fragrance, and ylang-ylang is purported to be an aphrodisiac. Use an aromatherapy diffuser to waft the scent throughout the room. Gather lots of pillows to toss on the bed so you feel like you are floating on clouds. His eyes will be captivated with your beauty and his ears will be enthralled with the melody of your voice as you softly recite poetry to him.

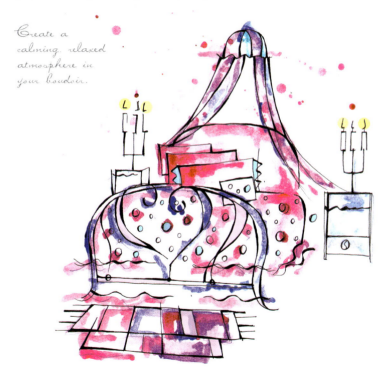

Create a calming, relaxed atmosphere in your boudoir.

reading and listening to poetry

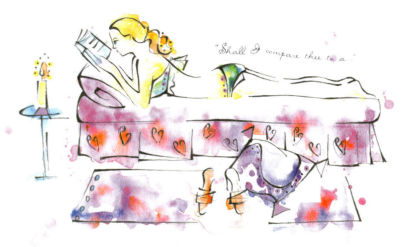

There is only one trick to reading and listening to poetry—do it from the heart. Aphrodite enticed and captured lovers into her magical web by the way she read poetry. It was said that men would leave her presence in a daze still mesmerized by her lilting voice, unable to function properly for hours afterwards. Poetry is pretty powerful stuff.

When you read a love poem, your whole body feels warm and tingly. No cold shower will quench your fire! Poems need to be read passionately. Imbue the poem with your own feelings. Don't be afraid to let its powerful intentions speak through you. Poems can bring tears to our eyes and set our brains abuzz with new thoughts.

Poems often require multiple readings, as they are laden with complex meanings. And they are meant to be read aloud, as the sounds of the words often add to the meaning of the poem. Sometimes the sounds recall waves crashing on the beach or the wind whistling through the trees. Listen. Try different voices, vary your speed, or stress different words. Does this change the poem's message? Think about the possible symbolism of each line. Sometimes a word or line refers to something other than what's explicitly stated.

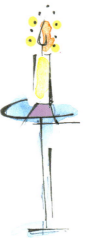

Yes, poetry is intense! But it's nothing a Goddess like you can't handle. How many men are lucky enough to have love poetry read to them? Give it a try! There might be some unexpected results.

poetry games

If you are looking for something lighter, how about some poetry games? These require more work on both your parts, as you will have to use your imagination to come up with clever rhymes. Everyone knows the old poem, "Roses are red, violets are blue, sugar is sweet, and so are you!" Why don't you and your lover come up with some new endings, or new verses, to this old standard? For instance, "Roses are red, violets are blue, I love it best when it's just me and you." Or "My toenails are red, your boxer shorts are blue . . ." You get the idea.

How about the two of you composing a poem together? One person starts with the first line, for instance, "I love the way you brush your hair."

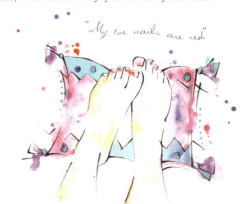

A response could be, "I don't know the next line, do you care?" See how far you can go before you run out of ideas—or are laughing so hard that you can't think straight!

Another way to create your own poetry is to pick a topic—a part of your anatomy, for example. Have your lover create a poem about his undying love and affection for your little toe!

Poetry comes in many forms, from serious and complex to lighthearted and silly. Dare to be different, Goddess, and experience all the varieties. Enjoy this adventure with the man you love. Who knows? You might have found a whole new world to share.

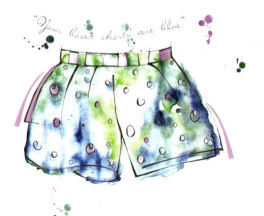

lights out!

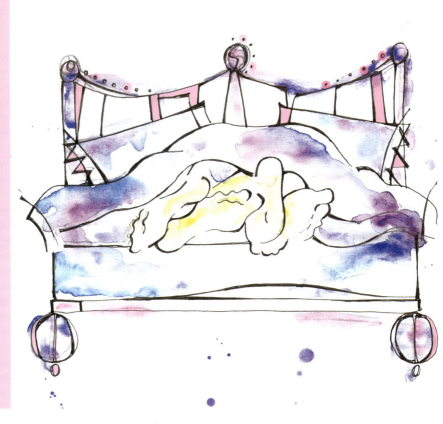

Your exquisite day is drawing to a close. Aphrodite would certainly be impressed! Look back upon all you did this day. It began on a relaxing note with your rose petal bath as you fantasized about the evening with your lover. Have all your fantasies come true? There's still time left!

What kind of love notes did you decide to send him? Have you filed away some ideas for future use?

You and your love can talk about the magical feast that you prepared for him and the sensuous fun you had feeding dinner to each other. Aphrodite would have been in awe of your dance of the veils! Ask your man what his favorite moment was, so you can be sure to repeat it at some future time. And what about that dessert! Yow! Ingesting calories has taken on a whole new meaning! And finally, reflect together on the quiet time you spent exploring poetry. Wow! It has been quite a day, Goddess!

You can take off your magic cestus now. You won't be needing it any more tonight, and it will only get in the way . . .

Lights out, Goddess!

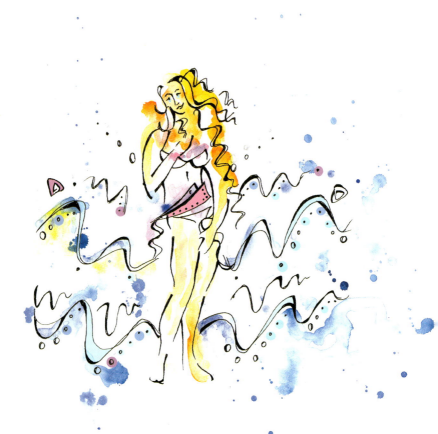